Anti-inflammatory and anti-neoplastic nutritional measures

Constantin Panow

Disclaimer

The author and publisher decline responsibility for any deleterious effect which could ensue from misinterpretation or wrong understanding and application of following text.

This booklet should not be considered as replacement of professional care in MD office or in a nutritionist consultation.

I0491138

TO MY GRANDPARENTS, FOR THEIR TENDER LOVING CARE.

COPYRIGHT 2020

"Let your food be your only medicine!"
Hippocrates (460-356 BC)

"Thus, Melzar took away the portion of meat, and wine they should drink; and gave them pulse.

And the king communed with them, and among them none was found like Daniel, Hananiah, Mishael, and Azariah; Therefore, stood they before the king. "

Book of Daniel, Bible, King James Version

CONTENTS

INTRODUCTION

Since Antiquity people have aimed at better health and well-being.

In our century of advanced science, we are experiencing a lot of difficulty distinguishing chaff from grain.

Our food is getting poorer because of overexploitation of soil and infested with chemicals.

Many people are turning themselves to bio-products.

This is not possible for the huge population of Earth.

I tried to resume in a few words well known facts about our health today.

Already medicine men of Old like Hippocrates suspected that all illnesses start in the tummy.

MODERNITY

Our knowledge has tremendously increased since. Health depends on an extremely precise and minute balance of Immunity.

We know that tumors are tightly linked to viruses, like Papilloma- virus for throat cancer, HPV 16-18 for uterus cervix carcinoma, Epstein-Barr virus for epi-pharynx carcinoma and lymphoma, especially Burkitt's lymphoma; HIV inducing lymphoma and Kaposi's sarcoma, to mention a few.

Hence, we presume that processing of food and content in our intestine is programmed at identifying Self from Non-Self, to eliminate last one component more efficiently.

Mucosal immune system gets confused if it is exposed to ingredients extremely near to Self in great proportion.

Then it considers body composition unhealthy and starts an autoimmune disease, nor cannot eliminate a tumor because it is also extremely near to Self.

Now you must know a certain percentage of gut mucosa gets sloughed every day, approximately 10%. Inflammation increases this ratio, of course.

LECTINS

This percentage is though highly variable, being dependent on several factors, and one of them are lectins in one's diet.

There are two ways of limiting amount of this component in bowel content.

One is by reducing input, that is cooking all ingredients which are rich with it or eating none containing it.

The other one is absorbing ferments, leavens which can reduce their amount, and on the other hand, help to degrade Self-proteins desquamating from bowel wall.

Daniel's Book brings testimony to the fact that you can live in excellent health on a purely vegetarian, ketogenic regime.

Many people, especially according to modern French cuisine do not cook enough their meals.

The result on individual basis is abdominal discomfort, but on a larger scale difficult to forecast, it may be one explanation for higher ratio of autoimmune and neoplastic disorders in modern society.

There is a huge amount of information about

treating different food to avoid lectins. Many people turn accordingly also to a gluten-free diet.

Plenty of cereals are devoid of gluten, and thus adapt perfectly to such regime.

STATISTICS

Statistical links exist between autoimmune and tumor disease, and many patients suffer both. MS is a good example!

GENETICS

Apart from that, we must consider that we ingest a huge amount of foreign proteins extremely near to our own body composition.

Genetically spoken all Vertebrates are tightly related animals. Pigs and all cattle are mammals (Triassic Period, 252-201 million years ago), remarkably like us.

Implanted cardiac porcine valves remain tens of years without deformity in human body. Nowadays diabetics use genetically produced Insulin, but for half a century commercialized hormone was of porcine and bovine origin.

Remember Moses would give precise recipes about thorough cooking of meat, already five thousand years ago! He also forbids his people pig meat.

Birds, which is poultry are related to Dinosaurs, (Mesozoic, 252-66 million years ago), that is reptilians, and thus much farther in Evolution.

With fish we have common ancestors among Amphibians (Late Devonian, about 363 million years ago), even farther away.

Shrimps and crabs are crustaceans. Clams and

mussels, as all those last-mentioned ones, like all Invertebrates (Paleozoic, appear about 3.5 billion years ago), are extremely far from our species.

Since more than half a century, medical workers have observed lesser atherosclerosis ratios in populations consuming a lot of fish. On average, they also attain an older age.

Legumes, like lentils and beans are an excellent source of non-animal amino acids. They are like proteins and are called protides.

Both ingredients need to stay in water overnight (Lectins) and be washed through a strainer next day several times before cooking (At least 1-2 hours).

MEAT DISGUST

Many people afflicted with a tumor become reluctant to consuming animal proteins, and especially meat: they find all by themselves the most natural way out.

Another food which supports tremendously neoplastic disease is sugar. By extension also Starches, which are Carbohydrates with an extremely high glycemic index (GI), should be limited to a minimum, if not eliminated, in a nutritional regime of a cancerous patient.

Such are understood as bread, pasta, rice, potatoes, and other cereals. They are transformed immediately into L-Glucose, white rice having a GI of 1, while Fiber-carbohydrates, possess a low GI, take longer to be processed in bowel and are digested into D-Glucose.

You can sustain yourself on Fiber-carbohydrates instead. This is greens and vegetables. Here, we come back again to the vegetarian ketogenic regime of Daniel.

You can easily adopt such a nutritional change. Your body would adapt itself rapidly.

Meat induces an inflammation in human body,

and its fat accumulates in a non-esthetic fashion in body parts.

Vegetal oils and fish on the contrary contribute to well-being and good-looking and possess an anti-inflammatory action on their own.

They contain Essential Fatty Acids, crucial for cell constitution and repair.

So, if you are fighting neoplastic disease, apply a vegetarian regime with a lot of vegetal oils. Switch different brands and origins to obtain all necessary Omegas!

Consume the oils raw and avoid frozen stuff either! As soon you heat them unsaturated acids are gone.

During the cold season you can eat fish raw, like Sushi, Seviche, smoked (Salmon for instance), but avoid such originating from warm waters, as it is infested with parasites. Those ones give liver cancer on the long run (South-East Asia being best example).

On the extreme side, you would be even better off on a Vegan nutrition!

A handful of different nuts would add also useful microelements and amino acids to your regime.

As a natural sweetener without calories, you can use Stevia.

BOWEL FLORA

Concerning food processing in small intestine, it is essential to provide it with a good flora.

There are many ways to do that.

Professor Gaston Turian in Geneva would propose during his lectures on Mycology during the 1970ties mold in rye bread.

People from Valais, a Swiss Canton in the Alps have had an exceptionally long practical experience in this field, as their rye bread was conserved for centuries in attics, constantly slightly covered with mold.

This population has been producing most successful skiers, strong athletes since long time.

Here should be emphasized that rye is a cereal with extraordinarily little gluten. Besides, such bread is called *Walliser Brot* (*Pain Valaisan*), in whole Switzerland.

Yoghurt, originally produced in the Balkans, contains Bacillus bulgaricus, an excellent germ to help digestion.

Similar can be said about mold in cheese, like *Vacherin Mont-d'Or*, *Gorgonzola*, *Bleu d'Auvergne*, but also about the white crusts of many cheeses.

Those should be consumed whole to have a positive effect on intestinal flora.

Sauerkraut is fermented cabbage, known already in times of Genghis Khan, and produced in many countries.

You can consume it raw, to be preferred Bio, seasoned with vegetal oil and Paprika.

If the taste is too sour, you can wash it in water. Do not throw the brine away, as you can drink it. Beware, it is laxative!

Other food which is fermented is wine, vinegar and strong beverages, preferably distilled ones, from plums, grapes, apples, pears, etc.

Those are only a few incentives to provide you with ideas about natural Probiotics, how to digest and process more efficiently proteins in your bowel.

Recent publications point to evidence of increasing neoplastic prevalence with high alcohol consumption.

One possible explanation could be that such beverages sterilize the intestine and reduce essential for health gut flora.

Hence it would be important to enjoy them only in moderate amounts. "Everything with measure!" says Philosopher of Old.

Current literature recommends one glass of red wine for women each day (1dl) and two for men.

If you suffer already a tumor, avoid such practice completely!

Apart from that, there exists since decades evidence about a link between germs, especially viruses, and tumors.

Resveratrol in red wine, grapes, and vinegar, combats them all.

Similar antivirals are Curcumin and Allicin.

Other companions which help processing and digesting our food in bowels are Pinworms. Their presence in number is crucial for balance of our Immune System and authority proposes Helminthic Therapy for Multiple Sclerosis for instance.

It is unnecessary to add them as a treatment. Every gram of earth contains hundred species of worms. Most do not survive in intestines. Pinworms do!

Every single human on the Planet has them in his gut.

Hence, it is sufficient to eat plenty green salad with one's meals to have enough of those pets at home.

With the AIDS and Covid- 19 Pandemics society experienced a huge leap forward in therapies of infectious diseases.
Probably near future would thus bring us many new anti-cancer treatments based on anti-microbials.

FASTING

Fasting has always been an essential part of medical therapy, which has fallen into disuse today.

Leaning down is also an essential part for maintaining good health and shape.

In many cultures this has also been a crucial point for centuries and thousands of years: For instance, the Passover for Israelites, fasting before Christmas and Easter for Christians and the Ramadan for Muslims.

This can be considered as an encouragement for us to consider how they were doing it.

BITTER HERBS

The Old Testament mentions bitter herbs during Passover. We can understand under previous consideration that this would limit appetite.

Those are many and you can find some in your own country without problems. The Middle East was especially rich with them.

Black pepper and other condiments also, above a certain amount, limit appetite.

Breakfast is the easiest meal to jump, and you can do this with a bitter black coffee (Bitter!) instead.

As children we would use sap of Pinetree as chewing-gum, which is bitter as well. It is also a bit sticky, but you can get used to it.

SALT

If sugars are promoting obesity, diabetes, metabolic syndrome, arterial hypertension, high cholesterol and neoplastic disease, salt is said to have an anti-tumoral potential.

Because of strong tendency to arterial hypertension in industrialized society, nutrition poor in salt is advised by medical practitioners.

But on one hand you would most likely have normal blood pressure with a vegetarian regime, and on the other hand you can use a preparation usually recommended for patients with cardio-vascular problems.

Such one contains Magnesium, Calcium and Kalium apart from NaCl. In France, you can find it from the brand *"La Baleine-L'Essentiel"*. In Germany between others there is *"Dr. Jacobs's Blutdruck-Salz"* available.

If you do not find such one in the wide distribution, your pharmacy will have certainly something similar to propose you.

Our ancestors were eating meat only a few times per year. They would kill the pig at Christmas and the lamb for Easter.

Many were suffering from Oxalate stones in kidneys and bladder.

Hence, it is important to drink enough on a vegetarian regime! Add a soup to main meals! Three liters per day of liquid is probably a good ratio, but you must consider expenditure.

RECIPE PROPOSALS

French type 4-courses menu:

1.Green salad (any kind lettuce would do)

2.Soup: leach and asparagus, half-half, seasoned with any palatable herb which you would enjoy.

3.Kjufte of plaice fillet (Or some other fish.): one bell-pepper, spring onions, which you pass in the blender first, then the fillet with dill, Arabic cumin, and sweet and black pepper. You separate with a spoon in small portions, which you cover with flour (possibly rice). Then you fry your Kjufte at medium fire. To be served warm.

Ingredients: 500 g fish fillet, 3 eggs, 1 bell-pepper, spring onions 2-3 stalks, dill, parsley...

4.An apple-pie, which you can replace by a quince-pie. This last fruit needs to be pre-cooked in a pot, before baking in the oven. (On a thin layer of paste, gluten-free!) Or else, a fruit salad.

TUMOR

If you are ill, you should be advised to take away course number 3 or eat it on a separate day (Not more than twice per week).

Replacement of course 2 and 3: Lentils or beans.

Those ones contain lectins and should stay in water overnight. The next day you throw away the liquid and wash them several times through a strainer.

Cooking follows seasoned with vegetables and spices to make the plate palatable for 1- 2 hours, at least.

You turn off the fire when you like the taste, or when it starts attaching to the bottom of the pot, which means the ingredient has released a high amount of carbohydrates.

Personally, I orient myself a lot after the smell, which the pot releases.

This means you need to stir the liquid at least every half an hour.

For both, apart from aromatic herbs, I add peppers and tomatoes. I start this preparation by frying onions on low fire until a slight golden color.

I season lentils with garlic, to be added at the last

moment, in order not to lose their allicin, and beans with onions which I fry previously.

After that, at table, everyone adds some sour stuff, either lemon or vinegar and vegetal oil. Last should not be heated to preserve its Essential Fatty Acids. Switch origins of those to sustain all needs of your organism.

As for green beans, I start frying them at low fire, with salt, and when they have lost humidity and have acquired a slight golden color, I add lemon juice.

ALTERNATIVES

1.Grated carrots, celery, red beets, which you can consume separately or mixed.

Tomatoes (Beware, unripe ones contain a lot of Lectins!) and cucumbers.

Seasoned with some acid (vinegar or lemon juice) and vegetal oil (+water, salt, mayonnaise, and mustard).

Spring salad: Ingredients: spring potatoes (boiled), spring onions, pickles (cucumbers), black olives, dill, salt, vegetal oil, lemon juice, or vinegar, mayonnaise, water...

3: Imam bayaldi, moussaka, sarmi, (with spring linden leaves, cabbage or Sauerkraut leaves, vine-leaves...) For these plates from Middle East and the Balkans, you can find recipes on internet.

DEPRESSION

Anti-depressive behavior should be stressed upon, especially exercise, and medical books advocate at least one hour walking each day.

Or, as Hippocrates would say: "If you are in bad mood, go out for a stroll, and if coming back you are still not happy, go out again!"

FAITH IN ONESELF

Last, but not least, to be emphasized is importance of optimistic mind and Spirit.

Many people have difficulty talking about faith, which you should have in yourself for the healing process to complete.

This one originates in confusion between Religion and Faith. First one is responsible for so many wars and dissensions, while second is a strictly private matter, where no one is interested to be involved in killing and even less so in destruction.

JOKE

And I laugh with my patients:

« La Religion est à la Foi, ce qu'est le Diable au Bon Dieu ! ».

PARADOX

One good example for this paradox has been Voltaire, philosopher, and writer (1694-1778), who had been living for long years in Geneva, and was well known for his anti-clerical inclination.

At the same time, he would say:

« L'Univers m'embrasse, et je ne puis songer- Que cette Horloge Existe et n'ait pas d'Horloger ! »

WEBSITE

I hope you enjoyed this short text.

I you have any questions or comments, you can reach me at:

www.thenopillshealthprospect.com